HARNESS YOUR CHAKRAS

ENERGY AWARENESS SERIES

ALEXA ISPAS

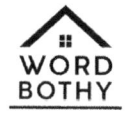

WORD BOTHY

Copyright © 2020 by Word Bothy Ltd.

ISBN: 978-1-913926-00-7 (ebk)

ISBN: 978-1-913926-01-4 (pbk)

All rights reserved. No part of this book may be reproduced in any form or by any electronic or mechanical means, including information storage and retrieval systems, without written permission from the author, except for the use of brief quotations in a book review.

Disclaimer: All material in this book is provided for your information only and may not be construed as professional advice. No action or inaction should be taken solely based on the contents of this book. Instead, readers should consult appropriate professionals before making decisions on any matters raised in this book. Readers who fail to consult with appropriate health authorities assume the risk of any injuries. The publisher is not responsible for any errors or omissions.

CONTENTS

Introduction	5
ROOT CHAKRA	
About your root chakra	13
Root chakra exercises	16
Chapter summary	23
SACRAL CHAKRA	
About your sacral chakra	27
Sacral chakra exercises	30
Chapter summary	36
SOLAR PLEXUS CHAKRA	
About your solar plexus chakra	41
Solar plexus chakra exercises	45
Chapter summary	52
HEART CHAKRA	
About your heart chakra	57
Heart chakra exercises	59
Chapter summary	63
THROAT CHAKRA	
About your throat chakra	67
Throat chakra exercises	70
Chapter summary	75

BROW CHAKRA
About your brow chakra 79
Brow chakra exercises 81
Chapter summary 85

CROWN CHAKRA
About your crown chakra 89
Crown chakra exercises 91
Chapter summary 94

Daily routine 97

Conclusion 107
Nourish Your Chakras 111
About the author 113

INTRODUCTION

We rarely live up to our full potential as human beings.

Often, we run on automatic pilot instead of participating in our life in a fully conscious way.

In this book, I will teach you how you can start consciously engaging with your life through harnessing your chakras.

How would harnessing your chakras enable you to live more consciously?

Your chakras represent the energies relating to the whole of your life, at every level of your being.

This goes from the most physical aspects, represented by the energy of your root chakra, to the most spiritual aspects, related to your crown chakra.

Making the most of your chakras on a day-to-day basis will enable you to tidy up your life.

Over time, you will decondition from agendas imposed on you by others, which are not in line with your soul's longing.

The more you consciously engage with your chakras, the more you awaken your innate potential.

This will allow you to grow into the person you were always meant to be.

As we begin this journey together, let me tell you a bit about how I approach the chakras.

My approach is somewhat different from most of the existing literature.

Chakras are often described as spiritual and esoteric.

They seem to be something to know about and marvel at with our minds, yet difficult to access with our bodies except perhaps through complicated yoga poses that are out of reach for most of us.

My own experience with the chakras has been rather different.

I encountered them through energy healing rather than yoga.

From the very beginning, I was amazed at how

easy it was to engage with them in my everyday life once I learned how to harness their energies.

What I'd like to teach you in this book is what I have learned through my experimentation with the chakras while working as an energy healer and through my own journey of self-discovery.

I will introduce you to a number of practical things you can do every day to nurture and harness each of your chakras.

In fact, I'm not sure 'introduce' is the right word.

A few of the exercises I suggest are common activities you may be doing already, such as the 'make your bed' exercise in the chapter on the solar plexus chakra.

However, throughout this book, I will show you how and why the exercises I am suggesting, no matter how mundane, can help you harness a particular chakra.

Understanding this will provide a depth of meaning to such exercises that you most likely didn't have before.

Once you understand exactly *why* you are doing something, no matter how simple, and all the ways the exercise is helping you grow into yourself, it is far easier to keep doing it consistently.

In addition, the more awareness you have of how an exercise serves a particular chakra, the more nourishment you will extract from that activity as you engage in the exercise.

Through undertaking the daily exercises, you will gain an embodied understanding of your chakras.

This will enable you to engage with their energy more fully.

By the end of reading this book, you will have a means of harnessing your chakras that is deeply practical and that you can easily integrate into your life.

I have kept this book short, so you can read it over the course of an afternoon and start using the exercises straight away.

If you don't know much about the chakras, don't worry.

I start each chapter by explaining what the energy of that particular chakra relates to before going into the specific exercises I suggest.

The first five chakras are closely linked to your body.

For that reason, the first exercise in each of the first five chapters is a physical exercise.

This exercise will allow you to 'switch on' the energy of that chakra within less than two minutes.

I then follow that physical exercise with two others that allow you to connect with the more subtle (emotional, mental, and spiritual) aspects of those chakras.

Your two upper chakras are already linked to the more subtle aspects of life rather than the body.

As a result, the chapters on those chakras only have two rather than three exercises each.

However, I have made sure these exercises allow you to get to the essence of those chakras.

My hope is that once you go through implementing the exercises for about a week, they will become second nature.

They will therefore no longer feel like add-ons to what is probably an already busy life.

Instead, they will become means to organize and simplify your life.

In the final chapter, I have outlined a daily routine that will allow you to integrate all the exercises seamlessly into your day.

And now, without further ado, let's dive in!

ROOT CHAKRA

ABOUT YOUR ROOT CHAKRA

Your root chakra is located at the base of your spine.

Its energy also connects to your legs and your feet.

I often think of the root chakra as the roots and the base of a tree, a ship's anchor, or a house's foundation.

Whichever metaphor you prefer, your root chakra constitutes the basis for your entire life.

Harnessing your root chakra on a daily basis is one of the best things you can do for yourself.

The more you consciously learn to engage with this energy, the more secure and pleasurable your life will become.

As your root chakra constitutes your foundation, the energy of your root chakra focuses on your most basic instinct as a living being: to survive.

An inner sense of safety is one of the hallmarks of a healthy root chakra.

Your root chakra allows you to feel 'at home' in your body and your environment.

It therefore allows you to relax in situations when there isn't any immediate threat.

This sense of being in tune with your body means you are likely to enjoy good health and vitality.

You are also likely to feel motivated to take care of your physical needs.

Your ability to find your way 'home', back to your roots, gives you a strong sense of trust in yourself.

Feeling safe and comfortable within your body and your environment is essential to maintaining a healthy root chakra.

It is therefore important to include daily exercises that allow you to achieve this feeling in an easy and consistent manner.

You are a unique individual, so what makes you feel safe will be different from the next person.

However, there are a few aspects that pertain

to the root chakra and that are fairly universal in making us feel safe.

It is these aspects that the root chakra exercises focus on.

As you read through these exercises, remember that you are the expert in how to best nurture yourself.

Please use my suggestions as a starting point for your own explorations into your root chakra energy.

ROOT CHAKRA EXERCISES

Massage your feet

One of the easiest ways to connect with your root chakra physically is to give yourself a foot rub at least once a day, or as often as possible.

Make the foot rub as vigorous as you can without hurting yourself, to get the energy flowing through your feet.

This energy will then spread the strengthening vibration of your root chakra throughout the rest of your body.

Try giving yourself a foot massage every day for a week and see how much calmer you feel, no matter what is going on in your life.

If you don't enjoy foot rubs, even simply

becoming more aware of your feet will bring wonderful nurturing to your root chakra.

Our feet are like the roots of a tree.

The more stable the roots, the healthier the tree.

Pay attention to the way you position your feet while talking to people and when you are by yourself.

For example, are your feet firmly planted on the ground, or are they floating above ground?

If you regularly wear heels, you might want to try not wearing them for a while, or at least giving yourself heel-free time.

Notice the effect this has on your sense of inner safety.

Bring attention to your feet as often as possible over the course of your day.

Remember to also treat your feet to an invigorating massage as often as you can.

Take care of your physical needs

Another way to harness your root chakra is to make sure you take good care of your physical needs.

This may sound simple, but be honest: do you always take your body's needs into account?

Whenever you take care of your physical needs, you are nourishing your root chakra.

In taking care of your needs, you are giving your root chakra the sense of safety and comfort it craves.

In return, your root chakra is going to reward you with a wonderful sense of safety that can sustain you no matter what life throws your way.

Here is a simple exercise I do to connect with my root chakra.

I ask myself, several times a day, a few basic questions about my physical needs.

Am I hungry?

Am I thirsty?

Am I comfortable?

Do I feel safe?

You can add any other questions relating to your physical needs that feel relevant to you.

It's amazing, when I ask myself these simple questions, how many times I realize that some of my physical needs are unmet.

I may suddenly realize that I've been sitting in an awkward position, or that I've been straining my eyes trying to read something with too little light.

Occasionally, I even realize that I am hungry and need to eat.

These needs are easy to take care of, once I articulate them for myself.

But if I didn't ask myself these questions, how long would my body have to put up with the discomfort?

Make sure you do all you can to be physically comfortable and ask yourself regularly if you are.

Your root chakra energy will flow so much better if you take care of your physical needs.

The more comfortable you feel in your body, the more you'll gain a sense of security within yourself.

This will provide a solid foundation for everything else in your life.

Tidy up your space

A third way to harness your root chakra is to make sure your living and working environments are pleasant to live in.

Our environment is crucial to keeping our root chakra vibrant and healthy.

The importance of feeling comfortable in our environment is often underrated.

Remember how I said that the root chakra gives you a sense of security within yourself?

The reverse is also true: your root chakra thrives in environments that make you feel safe.

You may initially think of safety in basic terms, such as whether the area you live or work in feels safe, or if your front door has a strong enough lock to prevent anyone breaking in.

However, that is only the first step.

I assume you already have the basics of such safety features in place.

If not, that is your first priority.

The next step is to make sure the environments you spend most of your time in feel as comfortable and harmonious as possible.

Think of it this way: everything you are surrounded by, on a daily basis, whether at home or at work (assuming these are different spaces), sends messages to your subconscious.

The problem is that our brain keeps us safe by prioritizing the negative over the positive.

As such, your subconscious will pick up on anything in your environment that might be perceived as a threat to your survival.

It will also pick up on things in your environment that are broken, misshapen, or in any other way not working.

Your subconscious deals in images and metaphors.

When your eyes transmit images of a broken lamp or a messy living room, your subconscious translates this into messages of alarm such as 'things in my life are broken' and 'my life is a mess'.

To put it another way: the environment where you spend most of your time, whether at home or at work, acts as a vision board for your subconscious.

If you were to make a vision board, you'd make sure it looked positive and uplifting, wouldn't you?

Well, it turns out you are always surrounded by a vision board: your living and working environment!

Isn't it worth making it the most inspiring vision board you can?

Look around your living and working environment(s) and make sure that every bit of it 'speaks' positively to your subconscious about the state of your life.

You may think that fixing your broken lamp, tidying your kitchen, or cleaning your bathroom isn't as important as your next work assignment.

But in fact, because such things relate to your

root chakra, they are the foundation for the rest of your life.

Take care of the small things in your life and your root chakra, as well as the rest of your 'edifice', will thrive.

One final note on this subject: the more you consciously engage with your chakras, the more your preferences may change.

Make sure you regularly ask yourself if your living and working environment(s) still match your preferences, and make changes as needed.

If you keep making changes to your environment that reflect your inner changes, your root chakra will continue to thrive day by day.

CHAPTER SUMMARY

- Your root chakra is located at the base of your spine. Its energy connects to your legs and your feet.
- This chakra relates to your survival needs and represents the foundation for your entire life. The stronger this energy, the safer you feel within yourself and your environment.

EXERCISES (IN BRIEF)

- Massage your feet. This will 'switch on' the energy of your root chakra.
- Take care of your physical needs. The

more comfortable you feel within your body, the more secure you will feel within yourself.
- Tidy up your living and working environment(s). This will reassure your subconscious that everything is taken care of and working well throughout your life. As a result, your body will relax and provide you with a wide variety of health benefits.

SACRAL CHAKRA

ABOUT YOUR SACRAL CHAKRA

Your sacral chakra is located around the area of your pelvis and genital organs.

Its energy also connects with the joints in your body.

This chakra easily becomes a storehouse of unresolved longings and frustrations.

In order to be emotionally healthy, it is essential to keep this area of your body clear of stuck energy.

If you do, your sacral chakra will bring a lovely sense of flow and flexibility into your body and into the whole of your life.

When you are connected with the energy of your sacral chakra, you feel there is more to life than bare survival.

Life is there to be enjoyed.

Therefore, one of the easiest ways of harnessing your sacral chakra is to make space for pleasure in your life.

What brings you pleasure?

The answer to this question is highly individual.

You need to engage with the sort of things that bring *you* pleasure, away from any conditioning you might have received while growing up, or in your current environment.

In case you don't already know what brings you pleasure, let's break it down a little.

There are different kinds of pleasure: physical, emotional, mental, and spiritual.

For example, physical pleasure can entail having sex or soaking in a long, relaxing bath, surrounded by lovely smells.

On the other hand, you may be more drawn to mental forms of pleasure, such as reading a good book or solving a Sudoku puzzle.

To harness your sacral chakra, incorporate whatever the word 'pleasure' conjures up for you into your day-to-day living.

It is also worth considering how you are giving

your sacral chakra a 'voice' in your everyday decision-making.

Given its proximity to your genital organs, which are the most sensitive parts of our body, your sacral chakra is your inner 'radar'.

Once you learn how to use it, this radar can guide you towards pleasure and away from pain.

However, most of us are oblivious to this excellent guidance system we have inside ourselves.

Its voice usually lies dormant within us, waiting to be discovered.

To harness your sacral chakra, you need to learn how to give your radar a voice.

Once you do, it will guide you towards those things that make your heart sing and life worth living.

SACRAL CHAKRA EXERCISES

Wiggle your hips

The easiest and quickest way to 'switch on' your sacral chakra is to wiggle your hips.

You can wiggle them any way feels comfortable to you.

If you need inspiration for how to do it, just watch a belly dancing clip online and you'll get the idea.

If belly dancing doesn't appeal to you, how about buying yourself a hula hoop and using it regularly?

Wiggling your hips is an easy and quick way to shake off any stuck energy you may have accumulated in your sacral chakra without realizing.

The sacral area is one of the most vulnerable parts of the human body.

It is so easy to tense up that area when anything uncomfortable arises in your environment, or even in your thoughts.

The more you can bring conscious attention to that area and keep it moving, the less energy will get stuck there.

Try shaking your hips at least once a day, even just for one minute at a time.

See how much zest for life you will start finding within yourself!

Do something that brings you pleasure

Another way to harness your sacral chakra is to make sure that every day, you do something purely because it brings you pleasure.

If that something also happens to have some other benefit, that is great, but that isn't the main point.

If you are not used to making time for pleasure in your daily routine, this might be the hardest task of all.

If so, do it just as you do homework in school: simply do it.

Eventually, you will get used to experiencing pleasure on a regular basis and will no longer treat it as optional.

Also, one word of warning: don't confuse pleasure with addiction.

How can you tell the difference?

By the level of satisfaction you feel afterwards.

When you do something that brings you pleasure, you feel truly satisfied afterwards.

On the other hand, when you do something that is addictive, you do not feel satisfied afterwards.

You crave more, and feel frustrated when you have to stop.

Make sure it is pleasure you include into your day, not addiction.

For me, especially while the weather is good, the 'something that brings me pleasure' is gardening.

I do it for the pure pleasure of it.

I delight in the smell of freshly dug earth, and enjoy witnessing the miracle of a seed turning into a fully-fledged plant.

I love eating the veggies I grow, but they are not the reason I do gardening.

I do it simply because I love doing it.

This kind of activity, that brings you pleasure without any regard for outcome, is a great way to harness the playfulness of your sacral chakra.

Maybe you already have an activity like that in your life.

If you don't, try to find what it is that lights you up from the inside.

It doesn't have to be complicated.

It can be as simple as watching the sunrise every morning or re-reading a few pages of your favorite book.

The important thing is that you make space for this activity within your day even when you are particularly busy.

It is also important you do not try to justify it to yourself or anybody else.

Though if you do need a justification for doing this activity, now you've got one: 'I'm harnessing my sacral chakra!'.

Do the 'yay' vs 'ugh' test

This third sacral chakra exercise is about giving your sacral chakra a voice.

If you do, it will help you make better decisions

and navigate your day-to-day activities in a way that brings fulfillment.

Before you do something, ask yourself: how do I feel about this?

Allow your body to respond, rather than your mind.

When you contemplate taking this action, does your body give you a feeling of 'yay'?

You might experience the 'yay' as an enthusiastic sound you spontaneously make, your body relaxing, or any number of pleasurable sensations.

For this exercise to work, you need to discover your sacral chakra's individual way of expressing delight in something.

For example, my sacral chakra tends to make the sound 'oooh' instead of 'yay'.

When I hear myself reacting spontaneously with 'oooh', I know that's something my personal radar is guiding me towards.

You need to figure out *your* unique way of expressing elation about something, that comes from your body rather than your mind.

Alternatively, does taking this action feel 'ugh'?

You may experience the 'ugh' as an unenthusiastic sound, your shoulders slumping, frustration, or any other unpleasant bodily sensations.

Just like the 'yay', your 'ugh' reaction is unique to you, and well worth discovering for yourself.

Let me explain why the 'yay' versus 'ugh' test is such a useful exercise.

You may not have much choice over whether you take this action or not.

For example, if you're working as an employee and you are asked to do a particular task that feels 'ugh', you may still have to do it.

But if every task at your job elicits an 'ugh' from your sacral chakra, that is useful to know.

It may take time to find another way of making a living, but you may need to do it sooner rather than later.

The more you do this simple exercise, the more you will benefit from your sacral chakra's intuitive guidance.

Just be aware that the more you do this exercise, the more vocal your sacral chakra will become.

Over time, you might notice that some places, people, activities, and so on always get an 'ugh'.

And then you'll know what to do, won't you?

CHAPTER SUMMARY

- Your sacral chakra is located around the area of your pelvis and genital organs. Its energy also connects to the joints in your body.
- This chakra relates to pleasure and enables you to shift out of survival mode into thriving, bringing much-needed enjoyment and restoration into your life.

EXERCISES (IN BRIEF)

- Wiggle your hips. This will 'switch on' the energy of your sacral chakra.

- Do something that brings you pleasure. This will harness the playfulness of your sacral chakra and allow your whole being to thrive in its positive, joyful energy.
- When faced with making a decision, do the 'yay' versus 'ugh' test. This will put you in touch with your inner radar, which can guide you towards activities, people, and places that allow you to thrive.

SOLAR PLEXUS CHAKRA

ABOUT YOUR SOLAR PLEXUS CHAKRA

Your solar plexus chakra is located in your solar plexus area.

Its energy connects with your digestive organs.

This chakra represents your 'inner fire'.

When strong and vibrant, your 'inner fire' keeps you resilient, helping you digest the experiences you encounter in your everyday life.

Central to a healthy solar plexus chakra is the feeling of self-confidence.

The higher your self-confidence, the stronger your 'inner fire'.

Self-confidence allows you to be excited rather than fearful of challenges, and to tackle them with ease and grace.

Therefore, to harness your solar plexus chakra, you need to grow your self-confidence.

It may help to pause and think about what gives you self-confidence.

You are a unique individual, and as such, you will have certain ways in which your self-confidence grows that are specific to you.

However, there are a few universal aspects of self-confidence worth pointing out.

One such aspect is that you are likely to feel more confident in yourself once you have achieved something, no matter how small.

Your self-confidence is also likely to be higher if you follow through with your goals.

This experience, of doing what you set out to do, is hugely beneficial to your solar plexus chakra.

It gives you a history of success to draw upon as you start a new endeavor.

'I got over that challenge, so I'm likely to get over this new challenge too', goes the thinking.

You may assume that you need to have phenomenal willpower to follow through with your goals.

This is not the case.

You will need *some* willpower for the purpose of maintaining consistency.

But beyond that, willpower is not the best predictor of reaching your goals.

The problem with willpower is that it is a limited resource.

It is therefore easy to run out of willpower and feel like a failure instead of growing your self-confidence.

In addition, willpower often comes at the expense of softer feelings that are important for your emotional life.

This includes self-compassion and the ability to have empathy for others.

If willpower isn't the key to reaching your goals, what is?

The answer is to choose your goals wisely, and from a place of self-compassion, rather than ambition and ruthless ego.

You need to set goals you are truly motivated to work towards.

These goals also need to be small and achievable enough for you to be able to reach them.

Do not set a goal that you do not have the clarity or the skill to work towards.

Only set goals that are within your reach using a small, achievable stretch.

By setting goals you know you *can* reach, that

stretch you a little but not too far, you'll be nurturing your solar plexus chakra one small step at a time.

In doing so, you'll be giving yourself the history of success you need for bigger, bolder adventures.

SOLAR PLEXUS CHAKRA EXERCISES

Adopt the super(wo)man pose

One of the easiest ways to physically 'switch on' the energy of your solar plexus chakra is to spend at least a couple of minutes at the start of your day in the so-called 'super(wo)man pose'.

This pose consists of standing with your legs spread a hip-width apart and your hands on your hips, staring straight ahead.

In adopting the super(wo)man pose, you are making your body bigger.

Over the course of the two minutes, this physical posture triggers hormonal changes that send out the message 'you are a winner'.

This activates the energy of your solar plexus chakra.

The effects of the super(wo)man pose were popularized by psychology researcher Amy Cuddy.

Her experimental studies show that our body language impacts how we think and feel about ourselves.

Our posture influences our minds as well as the energy we put out.

Amy Cuddy demonstrated the influence of what she calls 'power posing' or the 'super(wo)man pose' in a series of studies.

In one of her studies, participants sat either in the super(wo)man pose or in a low-power pose (leaning inward, legs crossed) for two minutes.

The results showed that those participants who sat in the super(wo)man pose felt more powerful and performed better in mock interviews than participants in the low-power pose group.

In another study, Amy Cuddy also demonstrated that power posing changed the body chemistry of participants, particularly in terms of hormones.

Participants who used power posing had an increase in testosterone and a decrease in cortisol.

Both these effects are linked with an increase in feelings of power.

Try adopting the super(wo)man pose for a couple of minutes at the beginning of each day for a week and see how much more confident you feel in yourself.

The more frequently you adopt this pose, the better.

Also, next time you have a meeting with someone you feel intimidated by, spend a few minutes in this pose before your meeting.

You'll be amazed at the result!

Make your bed

Another way you can harness your solar plexus chakra is to complete a task, no matter how small, at the beginning of your day.

The purpose of completing this task is to set yourself up for success.

Making your bed is a good example of this type of task.

It is an easy task, yet it can give you the sense of completion and satisfaction you need to start your day on a positive note.

'I only just got up and I have already completed something!'

That is a great thought to have at the beginning of your day.

There are two further benefits to making your bed.

For one thing, it will make your living environment look nicer, which is important for strengthening your root chakra (see root chakra chapter).

The second benefit is that when it comes to the end of your day, you have a made-up bed to look forward to.

This is a great image to reassure your subconscious that everything is running smoothly in your life.

This feeling of reassurance will allow you to sink into a deep and restful sleep.

If you are not in the habit of making your bed in the morning, try it out for a week and see how it works for you.

Hopefully you will love it, and it will become a lifelong habit.

If, for whatever reason, you find that making your bed is not something you want to do, find another easy task to complete at the start of your day.

Giving your solar plexus chakra some early

bonus points will do wonders for your self-confidence.

This will provide the foundation for a positive mindset throughout the rest of your day.

Set an achievable daily goal

One of the best ways to harness your solar plexus chakra is to set a goal and make sure you reach it before the day is over.

When you set out to do this exercise, you need to choose this goal wisely.

One potential hurdle in setting the right goal, one that strengthens your solar plexus chakra, is your own ambition.

We often set goals that are too far out of our reach, given our current resources and skills.

As such, we end up relying on our willpower to bridge the gap.

The problem is that willpower is a finite resource.

You only have a limited amount of willpower available each day.

If your goal is too ambitious, you risk running out of your daily dose of willpower before you have had a chance to reach your goal.

The result is experiencing a whole range of negative emotions such as frustration, disappointment, and shame.

All these emotions deplete your solar plexus chakra and could have been avoided if you had set a more achievable goal.

Therefore, the best way to harness your solar plexus chakra is to set a goal that, while stretching you a little, doesn't stretch you so hard you cannot reach it before the day is over.

You also need to make sure you choose the time to tackle this goal wisely.

It may be a good idea to work towards your goal at the beginning of your day rather than at the end, if that is when you have the most energy and therefore willpower.

On the other hand, if you tend to build up energy as the day draws to a close, that is the best time for you to focus on reaching your goal.

Either way, get to know your own rhythm, and make sure you allocate your best energy to completing this goal.

The more you make it a daily habit to set a goal, however tiny, and reach it by the end of the day, the stronger your solar plexus chakra will get.

You will then be able to rely on this energy when you need the confidence to take on bigger challenges.

CHAPTER SUMMARY

- Your solar plexus chakra is located in your solar plexus area. Its energy connects with your digestive organs.
- This chakra represents your 'inner fire' that drives you to take purposeful action towards your goals. This 'inner fire' is powered by self-confidence.

EXERCISES (IN BRIEF)

- Hold the super(wo)man pose for a couple of minutes. This will 'switch on' the energy of your solar plexus chakra.
- Make your bed as soon as you get up.

This will give you an early sense of achievement at the start of your day.
- Set an achievable daily goal. Prioritize your self-confidence over your ambition.

HEART CHAKRA

ABOUT YOUR HEART CHAKRA

Your heart chakra is located near your heart, in the center of your chest.

Its energy also connects to your thymus gland as well as your arms and hands.

This chakra governs your relationship to yourself and represents your internal soothing mechanism.

When you are connected to this energy, you can regroup and bounce back from the emotional difficulties you come across over the course of your day.

This chakra also allows you to connect with others, and to build a supportive and nurturing social network.

Your daily heart chakra exercises therefore need to address both your relationship to yourself as well as your connection to others.

HEART CHAKRA EXERCISES

Thump your thymus

One of the easiest ways to 'switch on' the energy of your heart chakra is to thump your thymus.

Simply thump the middle of your chest with your fist a few times, slowly but vigorously, the way gorillas beat their chest.

Take a few deep breaths after you do this, to further stimulate the flow of energy.

By thumping your thymus, you are activating the energy of your heart chakra.

This will allow it to flow freely and powerfully, and to spread loving heart chakra energy throughout the rest of your body.

. . .

Give yourself a compassion session

To harness your heart chakra, you need to set aside some dedicated time every day to process your feelings and do a 'self-compassion session'.

This sounds more complicated than it is, so please allow me to explain.

A 'self-compassion session' is a term I use to describe sitting with any unresolved feelings and allowing my body to fully feel them.

This initially creates some discomfort, as the feelings are usually negative and difficult to process.

However, the good news is that once I allow my body to feel them, the body is able to process and release these feelings within minutes.

Once this happens, the hurt caused by these difficult emotions is no longer there to build up into physical symptoms, self-sabotaging behaviors, or other ways in which unresolved emotions show up in your life.

Emotions that your body has processed no longer present a threat or a burden to you, no matter how difficult they were when they first arose.

It is probably best to set aside some time to do

this at the end of your day when you have a quiet moment.

However, you don't have to wait until the end of your day to give yourself self-compassion, if you need it earlier.

If at some point in your day you feel hurt by anything you come across, take the time to do this exercise.

Articulate what is going on for you and allow your body to feel and process the emotions that come up.

The more you get into the habit of doing this, the more resilient your heart chakra will become.

Spend quality time with someone

Another way you can harness your heart chakra is to take time to connect with someone in a true, heart-to-heart way.

Of course, there may be many people you interact with throughout your day.

But how many of them do you take the time to connect with on a deep, personal level?

What I am suggesting is that once a day, or at the very least once a week, you set time aside to connect with someone you get on well with.

Do this with no other purpose than spending time with them.

Is there someone in your life you can do that with?

You may find, as you attempt to do this exercise, that you have lots of 'purposeful' interactions with people, often to do with work or some other practical aspect of life.

However, you may struggle to find someone with whom you can connect in this way.

If this is the case, don't worry, this is common nowadays.

Use this as an incentive to find people with whom you can connect in a heart-centered way.

It will do a world of good to your heart chakra and bring lots of joy into your life.

CHAPTER SUMMARY

- Your heart chakra is located near your heart, in the center of your chest. Its energy also connects to your thymus gland as well as your arms and hands.
- This chakra is about the way you relate to others, which is underpinned by the way you relate to yourself.

EXERCISES (IN BRIEF)

- Do a 'thymus thump'. This will 'switch on' the energy of your heart chakra.
- Give yourself a compassion session. This will allow you to process your

feelings at the end of your day and release difficult emotions. Once you do this, the difficult emotions will pass. They will no longer be there to generate physical discomfort or become the basis for self-sabotaging behavior.
- Spend quality time with someone on a regular basis. This is highly enjoyable and keeps your heart chakra strong and vibrant.

THROAT CHAKRA

ABOUT YOUR THROAT CHAKRA

Your throat chakra is located in the area of your throat.

Its energy connects with your voice, your thyroid, and your ears.

Your throat chakra allows you to express yourself in the world, to bring yourself out into the open.

This chakra is about articulating your truth and getting other people to hear your side of the story.

Your throat chakra acts like a bottleneck for the rest of the energies in your body.

This chakra regulates the flow between your first four chakras (root, sacral, solar plexus, and heart), and your two upper chakras (brow and crown).

Your first four chakras are closely connected to your body, while your two upper chakras are linked with your mind.

The smoother the exchange of energy between these two areas, facilitated by the narrow throat chakra passage, the more coherence and harmony you find within yourself.

As such, the biggest challenge with your throat chakra is to keep it clear of stuck energy.

You can do this physically through making sounds and singing.

At a deeper level, the way to harness the power of your throat chakra is by getting in touch with your own truth.

This is easier said than done, especially in our noisy, fast-paced world.

Being drowned by other people's energies makes it difficult to articulate what you are feeling and thinking.

However, there are ways to find your way to your own truth.

The solution is to express your thoughts and feelings in raw, unedited form.

This will give you the space to explore what is going on in your inner world.

Doing so will also provide the basis for expressing yourself authentically in the outside world.

THROAT CHAKRA EXERCISES

Buzz like a bee

Here is a fun and quick physical way of getting your throat chakra into gear at the beginning of your day, or whenever you need to harness this energy.

I call this exercise 'buzz like a bee'.

Put your hands over your ears and make a 'zzzzzzz' sound with your mouth, pushing the air through your teeth.

Keep this going for at least a minute, longer if possible.

This exercise gets my throat chakra going every time, and I'm the quiet type!

I have even done it sometimes before meeting people I feel somewhat intimidated by, as my throat chakra tends to get blocked before such encounters.

It works wonders to get me to break the ice, and then things get easier from there.

Try it out and see how it works for you. Remember to have fun with it!

Sing

Another way to harness the energy of your throat chakra is through singing.

When you sing, you open a channel from your sacral chakra to your throat.

This channel vibrates your entire body.

Sing as often as you can and allow your whole body to resonate as you bathe in the strong vibration of your throat chakra.

If you start singing regularly, you might also notice your general energy levels improve.

This is because your throat chakra is connected to your thyroid, which regulates energy levels in the body.

Write your morning pages

'Morning pages' is a core daily practice of Julia Cameron's program 'The artist's way'.

This program is designed to help creative people heal their creative blocks.

However, this practice is so simple and effective that it can work for anyone, whether you regard yourself as a creative person or not.

The practice consists of writing three pages in your journal every morning as soon as possible after you wake up.

This exercise allows you to write down whatever is looking for expression in you.

There are no rules as to what you write.

The point is to write anything that comes to mind, exactly as it comes to you.

Do not think about it or edit, simply write it down.

I can tell you from personal experience that this exercise works wonders for your throat chakra.

This chakra benefits from being able to say what comes to you, exactly as it comes to you.

This is of course tricky during our daily interactions with others.

We often edit what we say to avoid offending people, hurting them, or causing unnecessary friction.

And yet, our throat chakra requires us to be completely honest.

This exercise allows you to fulfill your throat chakra's need for complete honesty in a way that does not damage your relationship with others.

Expressing your truth to yourself in this way gives you the opportunity to take a step back and gain perspective.

If you do need to stand your ground with someone, doing your morning pages will allow you to process your emotions before you address this person.

This will help you express your truth to them in a coherent, articulate manner.

The 'morning pages' exercise also allows you to give expression to messages from your subconscious that come up during sleep.

These messages are an excellent source of guidance and well worth examining in more detail.

This exercise also offers you the opportunity to give initial voice to half-baked ideas you don't yet know how to articulate.

Once you write them down, you will be in a better position to understand their meaning and express them in a more coherent way.

It is also worth noting that you do not have to stick to Julia Cameron's rules.

If the exercise appeals to you in principle but certain aspects do not appeal, you can adapt it to suit your needs.

I encourage you to find your own way of writing your 'morning pages'.

Try writing them at different times during your day, typing instead of writing by hand, maybe even speaking into a voice recorder.

Experiment and see what works best for you, but do give this practice a try, your throat chakra will thank you for it.

CHAPTER SUMMARY

- Your throat chakra is located in the area of your throat. Its energy connects with your voice, your thyroid, and your ears.
- This chakra allows you to connect with your truth and bring it out into the world.

EXERCISES (IN BRIEF)

- Buzz like a bee. This will 'switch on' the energy of your throat chakra.
- Sing. This will clear your throat chakra of stuck energy and allow it to act as a

channel between your lower and upper chakras.

- Write your 'morning pages'. This will help you give expression to anything you cannot directly express to others. This exercise also allows you to become aware of any guidance coming from your subconscious and give voice to your half-baked ideas. It provides an outlet for any of your thoughts, no matter how vague, and gives you the opportunity to examine them in more detail.

BROW CHAKRA

ABOUT YOUR BROW CHAKRA

Your brow chakra, also called your 'third eye', is located between your eyebrows.

This chakra connects with your eyes and your brain.

Given its alternative name, 'third eye', you can probably tell that this chakra is about more than your physical eyesight.

It is about your ability to envision the future and gain insight into the past.

Your brow chakra allows you to explore possibilities long before they become reality.

As this chakra is linked to your brain, it also provides energy for planning and linear thinking.

Through lighting up the path ahead, your brow chakra allows you to see, ahead of time, what actions you need to take to turn desirable possibilities into reality.

Your brow chakra also allows you to take advantage of your past experiences.

For example, it allows you to gain insight into what has worked well or badly in the past, so you can make better decisions in the future.

BROW CHAKRA EXERCISES

Envision your perfect day

Harness your brow chakra by using your imagination to envision the day ahead.

We often use the forward-thinking ability of our brow chakra unconsciously.

This usually leads to anxiety-provoking scenarios running through our heads.

For example, we may think of all the bad things that could happen to us or people we love.

However, you can start taking conscious control of your brow chakra's ability to envision possible futures.

Use your brow chakra positively by taking some time every morning to envision your perfect day.

For example, if you have a meeting that day, envision every detail of that meeting going as well as it can possibly go.

What would that look like?

Also envision other aspects of your day in advance, such as the great breakfast you will have, or the walk you might take in the afternoon.

Don't forget to envision the way you will achieve the goal you are setting yourself as part of your work on the solar plexus chakra.

Also envision the great heart-to-heart you will have with a loved one as part of your work on the heart chakra.

Put as much detail into your envisioning as you can and make it positive.

And importantly, envision your perfect day as if it has already happened.

This sets up your subconscious to look for ways of turning your vision into reality.

Delight in the achievement of this perfect day and allow yourself to feel the joy in every cell of your body.

The more you do this, the more you will attract positive things happening during your actual day once it gets going.

. . .

Identify your negative patterns

Another way you can harness your brow chakra is to identify your negative patterns.

This will allow you to stop doing the things that set these patterns into motion.

For example, you might identify the following pattern: every time you eat a sugary snack, you experience a sugar crash later.

This makes you feel lethargic and unmotivated.

To improve your mood, you impulsively buy something online that you do not actually need.

Following the impulse buy, you experience buyer's remorse, which further compounds your negative mood.

In an attempt to distract yourself, you watch something mindless on TV.

However, you find that your low mood is still there once the program is over.

Eventually, you find yourself falling into a fitful, restless sleep and wake up groggy the next morning.

By identifying this pattern, next time you crave a sugary snack, you have a choice.

You can either go through with this sequence again, or you can eat a low-sugar alternative.

Even if you do go through with your negative pattern, you are now going through it with more awareness than before.

This will make you feel uncomfortable.

Eventually, the discomfort will motivate you to seek an alternative.

That will make a huge difference to your life.

It is important to adopt the attitude of a neutral observer when identifying negative patterns, rather than resorting to self-criticism.

Identifying a negative pattern is already a difficult emotional experience.

Don't make it harder on yourself than it already is.

Be kind to yourself while going through this process and simply observe what you are doing.

The more such negative patterns you identify and change in your life, the more you will benefit from your brow chakra's clarifying energy.

CHAPTER SUMMARY

- Your brow chakra, also called your 'third eye', is located between your eyebrows. This energy connects with your eyes and your brain.
- This chakra allows you to envision possibilities in your future and gain clarity on the best course of action.
- This chakra also enables you to gain insight into your past through identifying patterns.

EXERCISES (IN BRIEF)

- Envision your perfect day as if it has

already happened. This will send messages to your subconscious about what you wish to attract towards yourself.
- Identify negative patterns. Review your day to see where you can make better choices. That way, every day becomes an opportunity for learning and growth.

CROWN CHAKRA

ABOUT YOUR CROWN CHAKRA

Your crown chakra is located just above the top of your head.

This chakra relates to the most spiritual part of you, a part that many refer to as your 'Higher Self'.

Your crown chakra also has the capacity to act as an 'antenna' that connects you to the wider world.

You can use this antenna to tune in and receive information about your environment and your place within it.

It is through your crown chakra's receptive capabilities that many of the people who possess so-called 'psychic abilities' get their information.

However, this ability is present in all of us,

once we get into the habit of harnessing the extraordinary energy of our crown chakra.

Because of the strong connection between your crown chakra and your Higher Self, your crown chakra is an excellent source of guidance in navigating your day-to-day life.

You can activate this capacity within yourself by regularly asking for guidance from your Higher Self.

You then need to wait for the answer to make itself known to you in a way you recognize.

This chakra also provides you with the opportunity to understand the wider meaning of your life, and therefore to live with a sense of purpose.

CROWN CHAKRA EXERCISES

Ask for guidance

One way you can harness your crown chakra is to ask for guidance every day.

Use your crown chakra to ask your Higher Self, 'what do I need to know right now?'

After you have asked the question, simply notice what comes into your awareness over the next few minutes or hours.

The answer may come visually, while you are browsing the internet or reading a book.

Or you may hear, sense, or 'know' the answer.

If you are new to asking for guidance, you may be taken by surprise the first time you receive an answer.

Your mind may throw doubts your way.

You may ask yourself, 'can it really be this simple?'

Yes, we all have this guidance system within us.

Once you learn how to use this process, you won't want to live without it.

Ask, simply ask, and trust that the answer will come in a way you will recognize.

Look for meaning

Another way to harness your crown chakra is to ask yourself, 'how does what I am currently engaged in fit into the bigger picture of my life?'

Take time to find the meaning in your current activity.

Is what you are doing meaningful to you or not?

When you sense that what you are doing is meaningful, it becomes possible to navigate even difficult times with ease and grace, with your crown chakra as your guiding light.

By contrast, when you feel that what you are doing is not meaningful, it is like your body, your mind, and your Higher Self are on different pages.

If you find that what you are doing is not meaningful, ask yourself what *would* be meaningful to you.

That will give you an indication of what you need to change in your daily life to fit in with the demands of your Higher Self.

It may take some time and effort to make the changes that are required.

However, knowing you are moving towards something meaningful will give you the energy to do all it takes.

CHAPTER SUMMARY

- Your crown chakra is located just above the top of your head.
- This chakra connects you to your Higher Self and provides an excellent source of guidance and wisdom.

EXERCISES (IN BRIEF)

- Ask for guidance, such as 'what do I need to know right now?'. Trust that the answer will come in a way you will recognize. The more you do this exercise, the more you will be able to

trust the process and benefit from the guidance you receive.
- Look for meaning. This allows you to connect what you are doing with the bigger picture of your life. If you are already on the right path, this will enrich your activities, no matter how mundane. If not, this will help redirect you towards your true purpose.

DAILY ROUTINE

In this chapter, I will show you how you can integrate the chakra exercises into your day.

My aim with this daily routine is to give you an example of when you may want to do these exercises.

You can use this as a starting point for creating your own daily routine, tailored to your individual circumstances.

BEFORE GETTING OUT OF BED (5 MINUTES)

Ask for guidance for the day ahead (Crown chakra)

We will start with your two upper chakras while you are still waking up from sleep.

When you sleep, you are in touch with your

Higher Self, which is communicating to you through dreams.

Asking for guidance as you wake up is therefore likely to be particularly effective.

The more you do this, the more accurate and plentiful the guidance will become.

Your Higher Self will get accustomed to communicating with you in this way.

Envision your perfect day (Brow chakra)

Do this envisioning while still lying in bed.

If possible, try incorporating some of the guidance from your crown chakra into your visual journey through the day ahead.

AFTER GETTING OUT OF BED (10-20 MINUTES)

Massage your feet (Root chakra)

Give your feet a quick, vigorous massage.

Allow yourself to feel the energy spreading through the rest of your body.

Wiggle your hips (Sacral chakra)

The more fun you have while wiggling your hips, the better.

If it helps, do this exercise using a hula hoop.

Adopt the super(wo)man pose (Solar plexus chakra)
Stand with your legs spread a hip-width apart and your hands on your hips, staring ahead.

Say to yourself, 'I am a winner'.

Thump your thymus (Heart chakra)
Thump the middle of your chest with your fists a few times, the way gorillas beat their chest.

Take a few deep, steady breaths when you are done.

Buzz like a bee (Throat chakra)
Put your hands over your ears and make a 'zzzzzzz' sound with your mouth, pushing the air through your teeth.

Write your morning pages (Throat chakra)

This is an excellent follow-on from the 'buzz like a bee' throat chakra exercise.

Your throat chakra, supported by the other chakras below, will already be warmed up.

This will help you express your thoughts and feelings more easily in your morning pages.

Make your bed (Solar plexus chakra)

Give yourself the opportunity to complete this task before your day has started.

This will give your solar plexus chakra an early sense of achievement and set you up for success.

DURING THE DAY (IN WHATEVER ORDER WORKS BEST)

Take care of your physical needs (Root chakra)

Taking care of your physical needs includes remembering to eat food that is good for you and drinking water in small sips throughout the day to keep yourself well hydrated.

Also remember to take care of your body's need to move and stretch between activities, especially if you sit down a lot during your day.

Ask yourself regularly whether your physical

needs are met and make adjustments when needed.

Tidy up your space (Root chakra)

Try not to allow things to pile up in your space, such as dirty dishes, dust, or general clutter.

A little organizing, filing, or cleaning here and there means that your environment will always send out positive messages to your subconscious.

This will allow your body to relax and provide you with a sense of health and well-being.

Do something that brings you pleasure (Sacral chakra)

Allow yourself to do this activity during your day, even during busy times.

You may find it helpful to put this activity in your schedule, to make sure it does not slip your mind.

Do the 'yay' vs 'ugh' test (Sacral chakra)

When you are faced with a decision, ask yourself: does this feel 'yay' or 'ugh'?

Allow your body to answer this question, not your mind.

Pay attention to the sounds of pleasure and displeasure you make instinctively, before you have had the chance to think about your reaction.

This will make it harder for your mind to override your gut feeling or your heart.

Doing things you feel passionate about at a visceral level will generally lead to positive long-term outcomes.

Keep paying attention to your radar and to the guidance it is offering you throughout your day.

Set an achievable goal (Solar plexus chakra)

When setting this daily goal, prioritize your self-confidence over your ambition.

By reaching a small, achievable goal before the end of the day, you will give yourself the confidence that you are able to accomplish what you set out to do.

This will enable you to make faster progress long-term than goals that are difficult to achieve and carry the risk of failure.

. . .

Spend quality time with someone (Heart chakra)

The point of this exercise is to make at least one of your social interactions purely about the connection with the other person.

Put such interactions into your schedule if necessary, so you make sure to have time for them.

Sing (Throat chakra)

Don't worry about how good your voice is, or whether you are in tune or not.

Singing is tremendously beneficial no matter how good a singer you are.

If you do not want to sing, you can gain similar benefits through humming.

BEFORE GOING TO SLEEP (10-20 MINUTES)

Identify your negative patterns (Brow chakra)

Go through your day and see if you can identify moments when you did something that set up a pattern in motion.

Then assess if that pattern is good for you.

If it isn't, ask yourself how you could change the pattern by replacing the initiating action.

. . .

Give yourself a compassion session (Heart chakra)

As you go through your day, you will probably find certain aspects that bother you emotionally.

This may be something that hurt you or made you anxious.

Allow yourself time at the end of your day to process your feelings relating to what is bothering you.

If anything remains unresolved, ask for guidance through your dreams.

This may provide you with ways to transmute uncomfortable feelings into something positive and productive.

Look for meaning in your daily activities (Crown chakra)

Identify all the ways you found meaning throughout your day.

This could be either in the activities you did, and/or in what you learned through doing them.

If the day felt meaningless, ask yourself what would need to change in your life to bring in a sense of meaning.

. . .

Ask for guidance through your dreams (Crown chakra)

As you are about to drift off to sleep, ask for guidance through your dreams.

That way, you will be able to fall asleep knowing that you will get answers to any elements of your day that still feel unclear.

CONCLUSION

Congratulations on reaching the end of this book!

The fact you have reached this point in the book shows you are truly committed to restructuring your life and getting more connected with the person you truly are.

By learning how to engage with your chakras on a day-to-day basis, you have chosen one of the fastest yet most effective paths towards personal transformation.

As you can probably tell by now, there is an exquisite order to the way the chakras build upon one other and blend their energies to cover the whole of life.

When you consciously engage with these principles of order on a regular basis, you cannot help but be shaped by them.

It goes without saying that the more authentic and coherent you become within yourself, the more your external life will gradually begin to match that.

Everything that brings chaos and confusion will gradually start melting away.

Before I say goodbye, let me just add a couple more important points that may come in handy as you keep following this journey.

Firstly, I encourage you to tailor all the practices I have suggested, as well as the order I have proposed in the final chapter, specifically to you and your particular life circumstances.

If the exercises resonate with you, and you can easily integrate them into your life, that is great.

For the ones that do not resonate, I encourage you to devise alternative exercises that suit you better.

We are all unique, and what works for one person doesn't work for another.

Take the exercises in this book as a starting point for developing your own process of engaging with your chakras.

I hope you now understand more about your chakras and how they relate to your daily life.

It is the principles behind the exercises that are important, not the exercises themselves.

You are the expert on what works best for you.

The sooner you take ownership of your expertise, the closer you are to connecting with your true Self.

The second piece of advice I would like to add is about the importance of consistency.

Engaging with your chakras is a continuous process that you must go through again and again.

The more you go through this process, the more you align with that deeply intuitive part of you, your Higher Self.

When you become able to honor all the different parts of yourself represented by the chakras, your life will start flowing smoothly.

Everything will be in good order and working harmoniously together.

I wish you all the best in your journey of transformation.

I would like to ask you for a small favor.

Reviews are the best way to spread the word about this book.

If you have found this book helpful, it would mean a lot to me if you could leave a review.

Even if you only write a sentence or two, it will help. Thank you!

NOURISH YOUR CHAKRAS

Chakras are well-known for leading to deep personal transformation, but do you know how to take care of yours?

In *Nourish Your Chakras*, energy healer Alexa Ispas teaches you one simple thing you can do to look after each of your chakras every day.

Download for free when you sign up to Alexa's newsletter at

www.alexaispas.com/newsletter

ABOUT THE AUTHOR

Alexa Ispas holds a PhD in psychology from the University of Edinburgh and had originally planned to become an academic.

A series of unexpected events led her to experience energy healing.

This extraordinary form of healing had a profound impact on her perception of the world and her place within it.

Becoming aware of the way her energy functions provided Alexa with a filter through which she could evaluate and transform every aspect of her life.

Over the next several years, Alexa trained and worked as an energy healer.

During this time, she used her psychology background to develop a practical and down-to-earth approach to energy work.

This approach forms the basis for the books in her *Energy Awareness Series*.

The series aims to help readers at all levels

understand how their energy works and how to interact with the subtle dimension of life.

If you'd like to stay in touch with Alexa and learn more about energy awareness, please sign up to her newsletter.

As a small 'thank you', you will receive a free book when you sign up.

You can sign up to the newsletter and receive your free book at

www.alexaispas.com/newsletter

Printed in Great Britain
by Amazon